3702923726

HEALTH, SAFETY AND SECURITY

in leisure and tourism

ANA BISHOP

PROJECT MANAGER: JOHN EDMONDS
PROJECT CONSULTANT: DEBBIE BETTERIDGE

OXSTALLS LEARNING CENTRE
UNIVERSITY OF GLOUCESTERSHIRE
Oxstalls Lane
Gloucester GL2 9HW
Tel: 01242 715100

D0994678

Hodder & Stoughton
A MEMBER OF THE HODDER HEADLINE GROUP

Acknowledgements

Compiling information for the two case studies presented in this book involved interviewing a number of senior managers in depth about the understandably 'sensitive' topic of their health, safety and security arrangements. Nevertheless, both organisations welcomed me with more than generous openness, so I should like to gratefully thank Peter Walker and Claire Hamer at The Big Pit, Blaenafon and David Williams and Rob Phillips at Thorpe Park.

Crown copyright is reproduced with the permission of The Controller of Her Majesty's Stationery Office.

Orders: please contact Bookpoint Ltd, 39 Milton Park, Abingdon, Oxon OX14 4TD. Telephone: (44) 01235 400414, Fax: (44) 01235 400454. Lines are open from 9.00 - 6.00, Monday to Saturday, with a 24 hour message answering service. Email address: orders@bookpoint.co.uk

British Library Cataloguing in Publication Data
Health, safety and security in leisure & tourism. – (Hodder GNVQ. Leisure & tourism in action)
1. Tourist trade – Great Britain – Security measures
2. Leisure industry – Great Britain – Security measures
3. Tourist trade – Great Britain – Health aspects 4. Leisure industry – Great Britain – Health aspects 5. Tourist trade – Great Britain – Safety measures 6. Leisure industry – Great Britain – Safety measures
338.4'791'0684

ISBN 0 340 65841 X

First published 1997

Impression number	10	9	8	7	6	5	4	3	2
Year	2004	2003	2002	2001	2000	1999	1998		

Copyright © 1997 Ana Bishop

All rights reserved. No part of this publication may be reproduced or transmitted in any form or by any means, electronic or mechanical, including photocopy, recording, or any information storage and retrieval system, without permission in writing from the publisher or under licence from the Copyright Licensing Agency Limited. Further details of such licences (for reprographic reproduction) may be obtained from the Copyright Licensing Agency Limited, of 90 Tottenham Court Road, London W1P 9HE.

Typeset by Wearset, Boldon, Tyne & Wear.
Printed in Great Britain for Hodder & Stoughton Educational, a division of Hodder Headline Plc, 338 Euston Road, London NW1 3BH by Scotprint Ltd, Musselburgh, Scotland.

Contents

Assessment Matrix

The tasks contained in this book will generate the evidence indicators of each element of Unit 7: *Health, Safety and Security in Leisure and Tourism*, part of the Advanced GNVQ in Leisure and Tourism (1995 specifications). They also meet performance criteria of the Key Skills elements indicated (the term Key Skills is used instead of Core Skills throughout – element numbers refer to 1995 specifications).

Students may provide evidence to meet grading themes through each task. All tasks involve complex activities and can generate evidence at Distinction level.

Key Skills Hint boxes precede certain tasks to give help and guidance on the particular skill developed through the task.

		Key Skills		
Task	**Unit 7**	**Application of Number**	**Communication**	**Information Technology**
Task 1	7.1		3.2 pcs 1–5	3.1 pcs 1–5 3.2 pcs 2, 4, 5 3.3 pcs 1–6
Task 2	7.1		3.2 pcs 1–5 3.3 pcs 1–3	3.1 pcs 1–5 3.2 pcs 2/4–6 3.3 pcs 4–6
Task 3	7.2 7.3	3.1 pcs 1–7 3.2 pcs 1–9 3.3 pcs 1–5	3.1 pcs 1–5 3.2 pcs 1–5	
Task 4	Review of Unit			

Introduction: Safe and Secure

Hopefully, all employers, whether in manufacturing or service industries, will voluntarily do all they can to ensure the health and safety of the workforce they employ, as well as that of their customers, visitors, or any other members of the general public. The leisure and tourism industry (perhaps more than any) is intimately concerned with people, their pleasure and their well-being. For this reason, leisure and tourism organisations should always pay particular attention to matters of health, safety and security.

The laws concerning health, safety and security at work today are extensive, and must be understood by everyone working in the leisure and tourism industry, both employers and employees. The regulations we shall be studying in this book should not be seen as mere targets to be met, but as the minimum requirements on which every organisation can build to achieve even higher standards.

SECTION

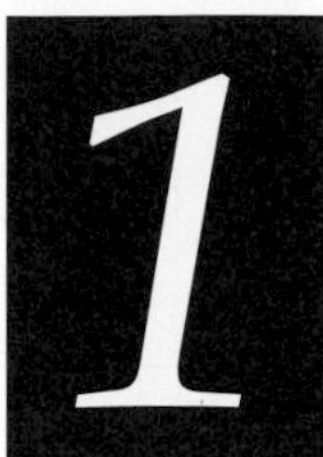

Health and Safety

Key Aims

Working through this section you will:

- be introduced to the structure of health and safety legislation in the United Kingdom
- learn about the Health and Safety at Work Act (1974) and its dependent Statutory Regulations
- learn how other Acts also influence health and safety issues in leisure and tourism

HEALTH AND SAFETY LEGISLATION IN THE UNITED KINGDOM

Figure 1.1 (see over) reveals that the service industries, as might be expected, 'enjoy' a lower rate of fatal and major injuries at work than agriculture, energy, manufacturing or construction. However this is no reason for complacency, for while some of these other sectors have seen reductions in accident rates over the last few years, the safety of the service sector has not significantly improved. It now contributes a larger proportion of the total number of workplace accidents as a whole than it did in the mid-1980s.

In manufacturing and agriculture the main cause of fatal and major accidents is contact with machinery. Like the rest of the service sector, workers in the leisure and tourism industry encounter machinery less often (there are exceptions, like fairgrounds and theme parks) which probably explains the lower overall accident rate. Nevertheless, this underlines how much care still needs to be taken when the leisure and tourism worker does come into contact with any item of potentially dangerous equipment in the office or on site.

Instead, slips, trips and falls account for about half of deaths and injuries at work in

	86/87	87/88	88/89	89/90	90/91	91/92	92/93	93/94
AGRICULTURE	145	169	158	150	169	157	174	180
ENERGY	336	289	308	260	246	231	203	180
MANUFACTURING	147	144	146	147	138	130	126	125
CONSTRUCTION	293	287	296	308	291	281	247	233
SERVICES	58	56	53	54	56	50	53	52

SOURCE: *Health and Safety Executive*

FIGURE 1.1 *Fatal and major injuries per 100,000 employees*

the service industries. It may interest you to learn that slips, trips and falls at work alone account for an estimated cost of over £800 million a year to UK industry. Accidents at work do not only have human costs, but financial ones as well. A recent survey (Health and Safety Executive, *The Cost of Accidents At Work*, 1993) describes the experiences of a transport company that lost 37 per cent of its annual profits through the costs of accidents.

Before 1974 **legislation** about health and safety at work, (such as existed), were scattered throughout dozens of **Parliamentary Acts** as varied and as contrasting as: the Boiler Explosions Act (1882), the Celluloid and Cinematograph Film Act (1922), the Factories Act (1961) and the Employment of Women, Young Persons and Children Act (1920). This confusing situation was considered by the Committee on Safety and Health at Work, under Lord Robens, which reported in 1972.

Largely as a result of this committee's findings, the Health and Safety at Work Act was passed by Parliament in 1974. The Act, quite simple in itself, was designed to provide a framework under which all the old laws could be progressively updated and replaced by new regulations intended to cover working practices in all types of industries in the United Kingdom.

It is important to understand exactly how all the new legislation is organised under the Act. There are three structural levels:

- the Act itself
- Statutory regulations
- codes of practice

The provisions of the Health and Safety at Work Act at first seem deceptively simple. It must be remembered, however, that the Act was essentially an *enabling* measure which was intended to: outline the basic responsibilities of employers; set up the **Health and Safety Commission** and the **Health and Safety Executive (HSE)**; give legal force to more detailed pieces of subsidiary legislation as they appear at a later date.

These subsidiary laws are called **statutory regulations**. Year by year since 1974, scores of statutory regulations have been introduced by the Secretary of State for Employment. They derive their legal status under the umbrella of the 1974 Act without the need for further recourse to Parliament, and outline in a more detailed way health and safety requirements for a variety of different industrial circumstances. Many of them are relevant to leisure and tourism. Usually, the statutory regulations represent European Union (EU, formerly EEC) directives which the United Kingdom Government is obliged to introduce into domestic law. Each new addition normally replaces, in whole or in part, previously existing British laws in a continual process of modernisation and simplification. However, the remains of the older Acts often survive and may still contain regulations about health and safety in circumstances relevant to particular industries. We should not overlook these older Acts as they may impinge on leisure and tourism operations. We shall see a good example of this in the case of The Big Pit (Pwll Mawr) at Blaenafon (see page 17), where legislation under the Mines and Quarries Act (1954) is still observed, even though the site is now operated as a tourist attraction.

Sometimes though, even the new statutory regulations are not detailed enough and in these cases the Health and Safety Executive produce **codes of practice**. These suggest, in simple terms, ways in which words like 'suitable' and 'adequate' when used in the legislation can be put into effect in real-life situations. Codes of practice have a peculiar legal status. They are not laws that have to be followed, but if a case of malpractice goes to court, magistrates or judges are able to admit any deviations from a code's standards as evidence against the accused. There are about 50 current codes of practice. In cases where there are no codes of practice, the HSE may produce booklets of guideline notes, which simply explain the law using less legalese.

Finally, the 1974 Act obliges the employer to safeguard the health and safety of two groups of people:

1 His or her employees
2 Clients and visitors on the premises, or any members of the public who may be affected by the activities of the organisation.

These two groups can expect exactly the same duty of care under the law. In the case of manufacturing industry, for instance a motor car assembly plant, there will not normally be many visitors, but at a leisure centre, airport or theme park, visitors will usually greatly outnumber the staff. The general public is often the primary beneficiary of the Health and Safety at Work Act (1974), although it is nominally written in terms of the employer/employee relationship in the leisure and tourism industry.

THE HEALTH AND SAFETY AT WORK ACT (1974)

The Act in itself is a very comprehensive, and necessarily, very generalised piece of legislation. Most of its principal requirements are summed up in only a few pages: these obligate an employer to safeguard the health and welfare of the people who work for him, and equally of any others who might be on his premises, or be affected by his business activities. They also define the duty of employees (and the self-employed) to take responsibility for their own safety as well.

The Act's main provisions are as follows:

1 Every employer has a duty to his/her employees, in that he/she must ensure their health and safety with respect to:

- the provision and maintenance of potentially hazardous equipment
- the handling and storage of materials
- instruction, training and supervision
- the physical condition of the workplace, and its access and exits
- the provision of a working environment free from risks to health and with adequate facilities for the welfare of employees.

2 The employer must co-operate with staff representatives or their trade unions, to develop policy and procedures of health and safety within the organisation, bring these to the notice of all employees, and establish safety committees if requested.
3 Employers also have responsibilities for members of the public not in their employment, but who may be affected by their

activities, either on or off their premises. Also, the responsibilities of self-employed people to ensure their own and other peoples' safety are established.

4 The duties of employees are not forgotten. Every employee must have reasonable regard for his or her own health and safety, as well as that of others, and co-operate with the health and safety instructions of the employer. It is illegal to interfere with any equipment provided in the interests of health and safety; it is also illegal for an employee to charge his employees for any health and safety provision.

5 The rest of the Act (the main bulk of it) consists of various legal provisions about the enforcement of all these new laws through the Health and Safety Commission and Executive, which is established and empowered. The Health and Safety Commission is a small panel which has the task of reporting directly to the Secretary of State on matters of health and safety policy. The Health and Safety Executive is a much larger organisation employing many people. It is responsible for implementing and policing the law in the workplace itself, as well as producing codes of practice, guidance notes, reports and statistical analyses, and generally promoting the greater awareness of health and safety issues at work. The Act gives the HSE the power to send in Inspectors, demand documents and evidence, issue certificates and demand improved standards.

6 Details of the offences that might be committed under the Act and the appropriate punishments are given. For instance, it is made an offence not only to fail in one's duties under the Act, but also to hinder the HSE in the course of its duties, to make a false statement to them, or to give false information in order to obtain a certificate. Such offences are punishable by fines of as much as £1,000 to £2,000 in a Magistrate's Court. In a Crown Court even heavier fines, or prison sentences can be imposed.

The Health and Safety at Work Act (1974) applies only to Great Britain. The situation in Northern Ireland is similar, but the legislation is empowered by the Health and Safety (Northern Ireland) Order of 1978. The wording of the Northern Ireland Order shadows that of the 1974 Act, and the dependent regulations parallel the British ones. The differences mainly fall in the detail concerning the enforcing authority, in this case, the Health and Safety Agency for Northern Ireland.

THE STATUTORY REGULATIONS

The numerous statutory regulations that have been introduced since 1974 are aimed at a wide range of industrial situations. Several of them are of particular importance to the leisure and tourism industry, and their essential requirements must be understood.

Management of Health and Safety at Work Regulations (1992)

This statutory regulation, which, like several others was introduced in 1992, became effective on 1 January 1993, and is intended to outline in greater detail the responsibilities of an employer to incorporate Health and Safety planning into the day-to-day routine of the organisation. It implements (amongst others) EEC council directive 89/391, and has an accompanying code of practice issued by the Health and Safety Executive.

All employers (and the self-employed) must assess the risks to the health and safety of employees and others as part of a continuous and on-going process. If there are more than five employees, the assessment must take the form of a *written report*, as must the resulting statement of company policy on health and safety. If necessary, experienced professional specialists should be called in to help make these assessments.

Having identified hazards and defined company policy, procedures must be established and brought to the attention of the employees, so that everybody knows what to do, and how to get to a place of safety should an emergency occur.

When assigning employees' tasks, employers should always bear in mind the capability of the individual to carry out that task safely, and provide adequate training if necessary. All health and safety training must take place within normal working hours. It is the duty of employees to report to the management any shortcomings in the health and safety procedures, and any dangers or hazards that they have noticed.

Special assessment of risks must be made with regard to pregnant women at work.

The Workplace (Health, Safety and Welfare) Regulations (1992)

These regulations largely replace and update the old Offices, Shops and Railway Premises Act (1963), and also implement the provisions of EEC council directive 89/654. The Health and Safety Executive has produced a code of practice called 'Workplace Health, Safety and Welfare'.

The basic environmental requirements of the workplace are outlined in terms of:

- dimensions (specified floor area and height for every worker)
- ventilation (fresh or purified; warnings if failure of system could be hazardous)
- temperature (must be 'reasonable'; heaters safe and thermometers displayed)
- lighting ('suitable and sufficient' and, if possible, natural; backup emergency lighting if needed)
- cleanliness (no accumulation of waste materials).

All workplace equipment must be well maintained and in good working order. Individual workstations must be conveniently designed and located with regard to emergency exits, and also provided with a suitable seat, if the work done there can be performed seated.

The floors and passageways of the workplace must not be slippery or obstructed. Windows and doors (especially if power-operated) must be safely designed, and easily cleaned. Stairs must have handrails, and escalators emergency stop buttons.

Toilets and washrooms (separate ones for men and women if required) must be readily accessible, well lit, ventilated and cleaned, and provided with hot and cold water, soap and towels, etc. There should be room to change and store clothing. Drinking water must be provided, as well as facilities for employees to eat their meals. Rest-room arrangements must separate smokers from non-smokers.

Personal Protective Equipment at Work Regulations (1992)

One of the best ways to avoid accidents at work is to ensure that employees use suitable protective equipment, for example: goggles and face masks, ear-protectors, chain-saw gauntlets, anti-corrosive overalls, etc. Unfortunately, there is no single code of practice to cover these regulations, which equate to EEC council directive 89/656.

After assessing the risks involved in a task, the employer must provide the worker with appropriate **personal protective equipment (PPE)**. The equipment issued must:

- fit well
- not impede movement
- be well maintained and stored
- comply to current UK or EEC standards.

The limits of the protection offered by the equipment must be explained to the employee, and training given as to its proper use. The employee *must* use the protective equipment provided. Self-employed people have the same responsibilities to the provision of their own personal safety equipment as employers have to their employees.

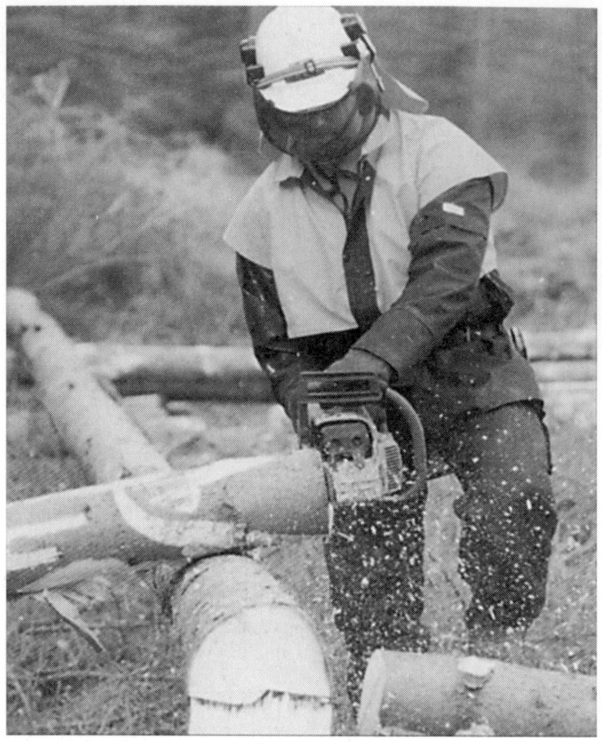

SOURCE: *Health and Safety Executive*
FIGURE 1.2 *Personal protective equipment should always be provided*

Remember that the same requirements that apply to the provision of PPE for employees also apply to visitors in potentially hazardous situations.

Manual Handling Operations Regulations (1992)

These regulations update previous provisions found in places like the Offices and Shops Act (1963) and the Factories Act (1961), and implement EEC council directive 90/269. There is no associated code of practice, but the Health and Safety Executive has issued guidance notes.

Quite simply, an employer is required to assess and identify operations that might require his or her employees to lift or manually handle loads in such a way that they are at risk from injury. Such situations might occur in an office as much as on a factory floor – boxes of computer paper are heavy! Having identified hazards, the employer must take steps to reduce the risk, perhaps by the provision of suitable equipment.

Provision and Use of Work Equipment Regulations (1992)

These regulations, equivalent to EEC council directive 89/655, oblige an employer to ensure that equipment provided at work is suitable for the purpose it is being used for, and that it is only used for that purpose. The equipment must be:

- firmly mounted and suitably lit
- well maintained and conforming to EEC standards
- if at all dangerous, only used by properly trained personnel
- provided with guards over moving parts or items that might fly out
- adequately provided with clearly marked controls (speed, emergency stop, etc)
- fitted with appropriate health and safety warning notices.

There is no accompanying code of practice.

Health and Safety (Display Screen Equipment) Regulations (1992)

Visual display units (VDUs) are now an everyday part of work in the office or factory, and present their own specific risks to the health, safety and welfare of their users. These regulations follow EEC council directive 90/270. There is no code of practice, but there are guidance notes available from the HSE.

Employers have a duty to minimise the hazards associated with VDUs to the lowest extent reasonably practicable by ensuring that:

- the screen itself uses large, well-formed letters, with no flickering and adequate contrast

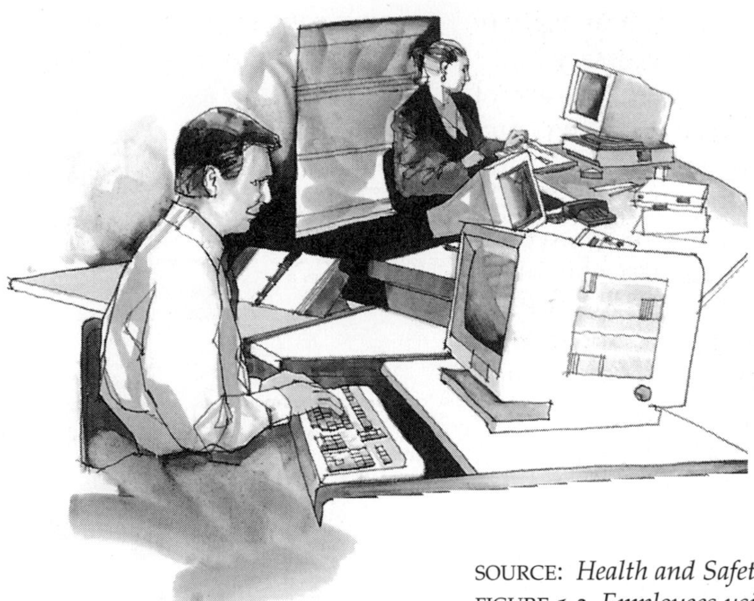

SOURCE: *Health and Safety Executive*
FIGURE 1.3 *Employees using VDUs are protected by the display screen regulations*

- the positioning of the screen, keyboard, seat and foot-rest should be adjustable
- the workstation should be of adequate size, the room well lit and ventilated (without lighting reflecting on the screen), and not excessively noisy
- radiation is reduced to a minimum.

The VDU operator must have regular breaks or changes of activity. To limit stress, the software provided must be suitable for the task and within the capability of the employee to understand. There must be no performance-monitoring without the operator's knowledge.

If the employee requests it, the employer must provide for an eyesight test, and whatever suitable visual aids may be prescribed.

The Control of Substances Hazardous to Health Regulations (COSHH) (1994)

The 1994 COSHH regulations replace those of 1988, and implement EEC directive 90/679. As well as a code of practice published for the new regulations, the HSE also has numerous guidelines and codes that were produced for the 1988 laws, but which are still largely relevant for the handling of a range of specific chemical substances. Note that lead, asbestos and radioactive materials have their own regulations independent of COSHH.

Do not think that these regulations apply only to industries like manufacturing, power generation or construction: there are many ways in which employees (and the public) involved in leisure and tourism can come into contact with controlled substances. For instance, camp sites may have to cater for large numbers of LPG (liquid petroleum gas) bottles. Swimming pools depend on the application of potentially hazardous chlorination agents. Many common cleaning materials can be dangerous and must be locked away safely when not in use – even in the office, some solvents may require special care.

The first step the regulations require is to identify substances hazardous to health, and assess the risks they present. This simply means – read the warning label! A bottle of ordinary washing-up liquid by the sink in the office rest-room is not a controlled substance if it carries no warnings, but a bottle of bleach almost certainly will be. If there are felt to be substantial risks from materials used at work, the assessment must be carried out by someone with knowledge of the health and safety regulations, outside experts if necessary.

The risks identified in the use or storage of hazardous substances must then be prevented or controlled as far as is practical, and (in the first instance) by methods other than the issuing of any form of personal protective equipment. If there is not a reasonable alternative to the use of the substance, then PPE is allowable but only as a last resort. Avoidable risks must be eliminated, perhaps by: sealing off areas to personnel not directly involved in the use of hazardous substances; improving ventilation systems; ensuring adequate washing facilities; limiting quantities of dangerous materials in store, and so on. Some listed substances are felt to be so hazardous that the regulations call for constant monitoring of exposure and health surveillance for up to 40 years afterwards.

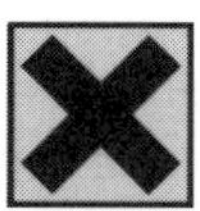

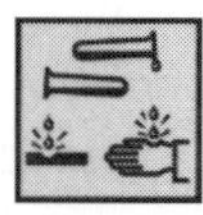

SOURCE: *Health and Safety Executive*
FIGURE 1.4 *COSHH warning signs must be displayed*

Finally, the regulations demand adequate training for all workers likely to come into contact with substances hazardous to health, and that the proper signs and warnings to be displayed.

Health and Safety (Safety Signs and Signals) Regulations (1996)

Most of the regulations empowered by the Health and Safety at Work Act (1974) at some stage call for risks and hazards to be adequately signalled with suitable signs. It is essential that warning signs are instantly recognisable. EEC directive 92/58 is aimed at standardising warning signs across Europe and forms the basis of these regulations. The

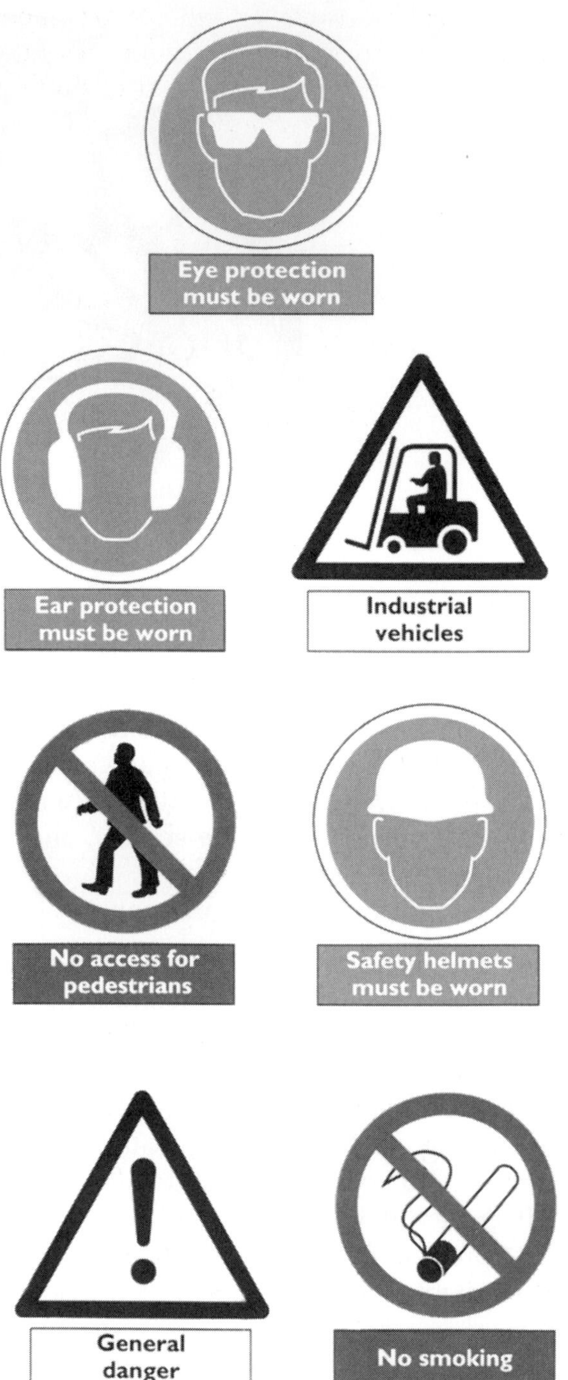

Eye protection must be worn
Ear protection must be worn
Industrial vehicles
No access for pedestrians
Safety helmets must be worn
General danger
No smoking

SOURCE: *Health and Safety Executive*
FIGURE 1.5 *Safety signs consist of easily identifiable pictograms*

law requires that employers display the proper warning signs as specified by the relevant British Standards examples. Although most of these consist of easily understandable pictograms, the employer still has the responsibility of ensuring that all employees know what each sign means and what to do when they see them. Fire safety signs and emergency exits are also covered.

Reporting of Injuries, Diseases and Dangerous Occurrences Regulations (RIDDOR) (1995)

Even if all the precautions required by these previous regulations are followed, it is inevitable that accidents will still occur. Every employer (or self-employed person) in charge of work premises has the legal duty under RIDDOR (1995) to report a fatal or serious accident to the health and safety authorities. A serious accident is defined as one in which a member of the public is taken to hospital, or an employee suffers injuries that result in over three days off work. Even dangerous occurrences which did not result in injury, but might well have done, must be reported.

The Health and Safety Executive or the local authority Environmental Health Department must be contacted by telephone as soon as possible after a death or serious injury at work. Within 10 days this must be followed by a completed accident report. The Health and Safety Executive collect reports from most industrial situations; the local authorities take responsibility for offices, shops, hotels, sports and leisure.

The 1995 RIDDOR regulations replace all previous legislation in this area. The Health and Safety Executive produce a short guide, which explains exactly what types of injury are reportable and what is meant by a dangerous occurrence, as well as a blank report form should one be needed.

Health and Safety (First Aid) Regulations (1981)

These replace provisions in numerous Acts referring to specific industries. The HSE produces a code of practice.

The employer must provide adequate first aid equipment should employees or visitors suffer injury or illness. A suitably trained first-aider must be present amongst the staff to supervise any treatment offered. The location of first aid equipment and assistance must be brought to the attention of all employees. The scale of the first aid cover required will depend on the size and nature of the organisation, and will normally be decided by mutual agreement between local authority inspectors and the operator.

Noise at Work Regulations (1989)

These regulations implement EEC council directive 86/188. Curiously, while noise emission controls apply to motor vehicles, they do not apply to ships or aeroplanes.

The employer has a fundamental duty to assess any risks that may be caused by noise associated with his activities. This applies as much to the managers of steel-foundries as it does to those of motor racing circuits or discos. The risk of damage to the hearing must be reduced to the lowest level reasonably practicable, before recourse to PPE. Two action levels of 85dB (decibels) and 90dB are stipulated, beyond which noise prevention measures must be taken. You may think these levels are surprisingly low – a busy street in a town experiences about 90dB of noise, the interior of an underground train about 100dB and a pneumatic drill about 110dB. Noise becomes painful towards 120dB, but long before this damage to the hearing can be caused, especially through prolonged exposure.

If employees are unavoidably exposed to noise above the first action level, they must be given ear-defenders if they wish to use them. Above the second level, ear-defenders are mandatory. Ear protection zones, clearly and correctly signed, must be set up so that employees know when ear-defenders are necessary. Unprotected personnel must not enter a second action level zone. The identification

HSE Health & Safety Executive

Health and Safety at Work etc Act 1974
The Reporting of Injuries, Diseases and Dangerous Occurrences Regulations 1995

Report of an injury or dangerous occurrence

Filling in this form
This form must be filled in by an employer or other responsible person.

Part A

About you
1 What is your full name?

2 What is your job title?

3 What is your telephone number?

About your organisation
4 What is the name of your organisation?

5 What is its address and postcode?

6 What type of work does the organisation do?

Part B

About the incident
1 On what date did the incident happen?

/ /

2 At what time did the incident happen?
(Please use the 24-hour clock eg 0600)

3 Did the incident happen at the above address?

Yes ☐ Go to question 4

No ☐ Where did the incident happen?

☐ elsewhere in your organisation – give the name, address and postcode

☐ at someone else's premises – give the name, address and postcode

☐ in a public place – give details of where it happened

If you do not know the postcode, what is the name of the local authority?

4 In which department, or where on the premises, did the incident happen?

Part C

About the injured person
If you are reporting a dangerous occurrence, go to Part F.
If more than one person was injured in the same incident, please attach the details asked for in Part C and Part D for each injured person.

1 What is their full name?

2 What is their home address and postcode?

3 What is their home phone number?

4 How old are they?

5 Are they

☐ male?

☐ female?

6 What is their job title?

7 Was the injured person (tick only one box)

☐ one of your employees?

☐ on a training scheme? Give details:

☐ on work experience?

☐ employed by someone else? Give details of the employer:

☐ self-employed and at work?

☐ a member of the public?

Part D

About the injury
1 What was the injury? (eg fracture, laceration)

2 What part of the body was injured?

F2508 (01/96)

Continued overleaf

3 Was the injury (tick the one box that applies)

☐ a fatality?

☐ a major injury or condition? (see accompanying notes)

☐ an injury to an employee or self-employed person which prevented them doing their normal work for more than 3 days?

☐ an injury to a member of the public which meant they had to be taken from the scene of the accident to a hospital for treatment?

4 Did the injured person (tick all the boxes that apply)

☐ become unconscious?

☐ need resuscitation?

☐ remain in hospital for more than 24 hours?

☐ none of the above.

Part E

About the kind of accident
Please tick the one box that best describes what happened, then go to Part G.

☐ Contact with moving machinery or material being machined

☐ Hit by a moving, flying or falling object

☐ Hit by a moving vehicle

☐ Hit something fixed or stationary

☐ Injured while handling, lifting or carrying

☐ Slipped, tripped or fell on the same level

☐ Fell from a height
How high was the fall?
metres

☐ Trapped by something collapsing

☐ Drowned or asphyxiated

☐ Exposed to, or in contact with, a harmful substance

☐ Exposed to fire

☐ Exposed to an explosion

☐ Contact with electricity or an electrical discharge

☐ Injured by an animal

☐ Physically assaulted by a person

☐ Another kind of accident (describe it in Part G)

Part F

Dangerous occurrences
Enter the number of the dangerous occurrence you are reporting. (The numbers are given in the Regulations and in the notes which accompany this form.)

Part G

Describing what happened
Give as much detail as you can. For instance

- the name of any substance involved
- the name and type of any machine involved
- the events that led to the incident
- the part played by any people.

If it was a personal injury, give details of what the person was doing. Describe any action that has since been taken to prevent a similar incident. Use a separate piece of paper if you need to.

Part H

Your signature
Signature

Date

/ /

Where to send the form
Please send it to the Enforcing Authority for the place where it happened. If you do not know the Enforcing Authority, send it to the nearest HSE office.

For official use
Client number | Location number | Event number | ☐ INV REP ☐ Y ☐ N

SOURCE: *Health and Safety Executive*

FIGURE 1.6 *The RIDDOR form must be completed after serious accidents*

of noise hazards and the use of PPE must form part of the employee's training.

The implications of this regulation to the leisure and tourism industry are quite profound. Many fairground, theme park and sporting attractions can be noisy, and the volumes associated with pop concerts and discos are often clearly in excess of the prescribed action levels, although seemingly socially acceptable. Legal responsibilities still exist, even if it appears that enforcement of the regulations is not generally observed.

Though not necessarily covered by the provisions of this particular regulation, a further problem concerning noise must be mentioned. All of us have a duty to ensure that what we do does not represent an annoyance to others. Noise pollution is a matter taken seriously today by Environmental Health inspectors, who have legal powers to safeguard the interests of those who suffer from a noisy neighbour, be it an individual that causes the nuisance or an organised event. If you suspect that noise from your activities could distress others, you should check with the local council before, not after, the arguments start.

FIRE PRECAUTIONS AND FOOD SAFETY

We have already noted that statutory regulations under the Health and Safety at Work Act (1974) are not the only items of legislation that have to be taken into account by the leisure and tourism industry in its efforts to ensure the well-being of its customers. Other Acts, for instance the Offices, Shops and Railway Premises Act (1963), survive in part, and may still contain clauses relevant to certain situations. Later, in the case studies we will learn how leisure and tourism organisations are sometimes subject to legislation of a very specific nature: for example, the Mines and Quarries Act (1954) at the Big Pit, Blaenafon, and the Merchant Shipping Act (1995) at Thorpe Park. However, the following pair of regulations, not related to the Health and Safety at Work Act (1974), will affect almost every leisure and tourism operator, and we must consider them.

The Fire Precautions Act (1971)

One of the most important duties of any organisation in the leisure and tourism industry is to protect both its staff and customers from the danger of fire on its premises. For the small operator, commonsense precautions about emergency exits, extinguishers, well-maintained and operated electrical equipment apply just as they do at home. But for larger premises, fire risks become a concern for the law.

Shops, places of entertainment and hotels all have size limits beyond which a fire certificate must be issued by the local fire authority. Its terms must be complied to on pain of heavy fines. The precise size limits that apply in different types of premises are a complex matter to interpret (buildings often have more than one use), and the best advice will always be that if it is even suspected that a fire certificate is necessary, contact the fire authority. A representative of the local fire brigade will inspect the premises, not only to offer the benefits of their very considerable experience, but also to ensure that: fire escapes and fire doors are adequate and are kept clear, staff are trained in matters of fire safety and regular drills are held, and that suitable fire-fighting equipment is provided. A fire certificate will be awarded only on compliance with all these stipulations.

A complete review of fire safety in the workplace is currently in hand, and important changes in legislation are expected from 1997.

The Food Safety Act (1990)

Many, perhaps most, leisure and tourism organisations supplement their income by offering the sale of food and drink on their premises, and since 1990, must comply with the Food Safety Act. While the precise demands of this Act are primarily the concern of the student of catering, we should note that it demands high standards of cleanliness and sanitation at all times in the preparation and storage of food. Local Authority inspectors have powers to enforce the Act by means of fines, and even the prohibition of the further sale of food. If alcoholic drinks are sold or consumed on the premises, a liquor licence is necessary.

SECTION

2

Security

Key Aims

Working through this section you will:

- be made aware of the need for security in the leisure and tourism industries
- be introduced to the laws about consumer protection, liability and licensing

For most of us, personal security forms part of our everyday routine – few people would think of leaving their front doors or vehicles unlocked. The precise level of caution we adopt, from simply closing a window to installing expensive burglar alarms and car immobilisers, is an effect of the danger we feel the local environment threatens. Not many people would willingly venture to a leisure or tourism destination if they felt that by doing so they were placing themselves in real danger of violence or crime. The fortunes of the tourism industries of Northern Ireland or Yugoslavia are obviously affected by perceptions of personal safety. A visit to a local school fête may be seen as a less hazardous family outing than going to many big football matches.

The managers of a successful leisure or tourism event or operation must make their visitors feel that their security is not threatened in any way while in their care. The precise level of security chosen will depend on the scale of the operation and the local circumstances. In an age when armed guards patrol British airports, most people will not be offended by a visible security presence, commensurate with the nature of the event. People have the right to expect a duty of care from leisure and tourism operators, designed to protect them against violence, theft of their belongings, sabotage and terrorism, or the unwanted disclosure of personal information about them.

In addition, employees in the industry are entitled to protection from unruly members of the public. The HSE publishes codes of practice outlining ways employers can protect staff in various sectors (retail, banks, schools) from abuse.

THE SALE OF GOODS ACT (1979) AND THE SUPPLY OF GOODS AND SERVICES ACT (1982)

The leisure and tourism industry operates through the supply of goods and services. The comprehensive legislation covering such transactions is designed to protect both the supplier and the customer, and both should know their rights under the law.

The Sale of Goods Act (1979) refers to 'goods' only, i.e. actual articles, not services or financial transactions. However, since many leisure and tourism operations involve some retailing, the fundamental requirements of the Act should be understood.

The Act describes the contractual duties of both parties when a sale is made, and their rights in areas such as payment and delivery. The best known section concerns the quality of the goods themselves; they have to be 'fit for the purpose for which they are commonly supplied ... free from defects, safe and durable'. If the goods are described as damaged or blemished in any way, and if the purchaser has had ample opportunity to examine them in such a way that he or she ought to be able to recognise their condition, then the seller has no further obligations should they be subsequently rejected. Simply changing one's mind about a purchase puts no legal obligation on the seller to refund or exchange goods, although some retailers operate their own, more relaxed, policy in this matter.

Under the Supply of Goods and Services Act (1982), the customer has a right to expect that the supplier shall carry out a service with reasonable care and skill, and within a reasonable period (if no time limit is fixed by contract). Put quite simply, the supplier of a service must be up to the job, or the customer can expect a refund. Equally, the supplier has a right to expect a reasonable sum in payment for the service.

THE CONSUMER PROTECTION ACT (1987)

Many older Acts were repealed in whole or in part when this Act became law in 1987. It works in three ways to further safeguard the interests of consumers.

1 The Act establishes the liability of producers or suppliers of goods for death, injury or damage to property caused to consumers by defects in the goods they have sold.
2 It becomes an offence to supply goods that do not comply to safety standards. The Department of Trade and Industry is responsible for producing safety regulations governing all types of goods on sale, after due consultation with the Health and Safety Commission, industrial representatives or other relevant parties.
3 Lastly, the Act stipulates that goods must not be priced in a misleading or deceptive manner.

PACKAGE TRAVEL, PACKAGE HOLIDAYS AND PACKAGE TOURS REGULATIONS (1992)

These regulations were introduced into consumer law by the Secretary of State for Trade and Industry in response to EEC directive 90/314, and after a spate of well publicised collapses of package holiday companies. They offer consumers specific protection against malpractice in the package holiday industry. The regulations require that brochures advertising package holidays must not be misleading, and should be clearly set out, with prices and other relevant informa-

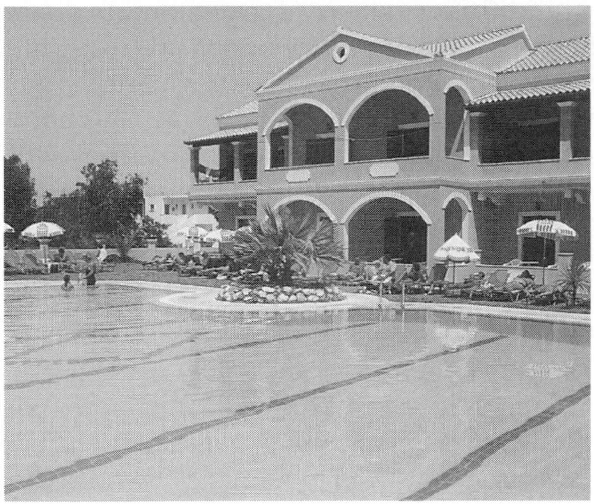

SOURCE: *Unijet, Greece and Turkey brochure 1997*

FIGURE 2.1 *An accurate depiction of the Unijet development in Corfu*

tion clearly displayed. The contents of the brochure imply a warranty for purposes of contract, and if the actual package falls short of what had been promised, then compensation must be paid.

Passport and visa requirements, as well as any health formalities (such as vaccination certificates) must be explained, as must the operator's arrangements for security of money paid and repatriation in case of insolvency. It is a legal requirement for the package tour operator to safeguard the consumer's investment in the holiday, through financial arrangements with insurance companies or professional organisations, so that if the firm collapses the holiday will not be lost, nor the client stranded abroad.

The operator is responsible for all aspects of the package including the services of client organisations, like hotels or airlines. Should the holiday fall short of contractual obligations, the consumer can expect a refund, or a transfer home or to another destination.

No last-minute price rises are allowed, unless the possibility is specifically agreed within the terms of the contract; no price rise can be made within 30 days of the departure date. If unforeseen events demand changes to the contract, the consumer must be contacted immediately and given the option of cancellation with a full refund.

THE CONSUMER CREDIT ACT (1974)

Holidays are expensive and many people will choose to pay for them by credit and the terms of the Consumer Credit Act (1974) govern the nature of the agreement. The Act stipulates that credit agreements must be clearly explained to the customer, and contain no hidden surprises that could not be reasonably ascertained beforehand. Even the size of the small print on the document is regulated. A 'cooling-off' period, during which the customer has the right to change his or her mind, has to be observed. There are measures to protect young people from entering credit agreements against their best interests. The rights of the provider to recovery of goods, or cessation of services, in the event of non-payment are also described.

THE DATA PROTECTION ACT (1984)

The sale of information about customers (names, addresses, purchasing habits, bad payment histories) is a fact of life in modern business. The increasing use of computer databases holding customer information has made this trade even easier. In 1984 the Government acted to give members of the public the right to know exactly what information was being held about them on computer files, and to have inaccuracies corrected. When requested, a company is legally obliged to provide a copy of any file held about an individual. A small fee may be charged. Every company holding such files must register with the Data Protection Registrar. Failure to comply with either of these requirements may result in prosecution. Perversely, there is no legislation covering files held on 'paper' systems, and the public still has no right to demand access to them.

LIABILITY AND LICENSING LAWS

Most people will already be aware that it is illegal to sell alcoholic drinks on a premises or at an event without a *liquor licence*. This is obtained by application to a Magistrate's Court. The local authority similarly issues a number of licences covering activities that take place at leisure and tourism venues. A *cinema licence* or a *theatre licence* will be needed for performances of films or plays, the former including video juke boxes. Sporting events held indoors in the presence of spectators require an *indoor sports licence*. A *public entertainments licence* is needed for concerts and discos and dancing at indoor as well as outdoor venues.

The issuing of a licence is not a mere formality. The authorities will take the advice of the police and fire service on:

- the suitability and safety of the premises
- the good character of the applicant
- any objections from local people about the impact to the neighbourhood.

The award of a licence has fire precautions implications, so the issuing of, for instance, a public entertainment licence and a fire certificate would go hand in hand. If, even after the award of the necessary licences, local people still believe they are suffering unreasonably from sporting, leisure or entertainment events, they are entitled to bring an action under the Public Order Act (1986). They will need to convince a court however, that the nuisance is not the result of a single occasion but is one that re-occurs over a period of time.

The operator of a leisure or tourism facility is made responsible by the Occupiers' Liability Act (1984) for the safety of his or her customers and any others who may be affected. If death or injury is caused by defective equipment or dangerous pathways (for example), the operator will be responsible under the law for compensation. If cricket balls descend on neighbours' greenhouses, it is the duty of the cricket club to make good the damage. Customers have the right to expect that operators in the leisure and tourism sector are adequately covered by public liability insurance against claims for negligence. Amounts awarded by courts can be extremely large, and no event should go ahead if the organisers are not sure of their insurance cover, both for public liability, and loss to themselves from fire, theft or cancellation.

SECTION

3

Two Case Studies

Key Aims

Working through this section you will:

- learn how key laws and regulations on health, safety and security apply to two contrasting leisure and tourism venues
- learn how other regulatory codes and Acts of Parliament influence their operation
- learn how these organisations cope in practice with the demands of the law

The two case studies in this section have been carefully chosen to illustrate the contrasting challenges they present to their respective managements. A wide range of potential hazards will be encountered, resulting in the implementation of not only the statutory regulations of the Health and Safety at Work Act (1974), and other key laws, but also more specialised regulations and some Acts of Parliament. Additionally, different approaches to security have arisen from the need to deal with small groups of less than twenty people in one case to tens of thousands in the other.

THE BIG PIT (PWLL MAWR) MINING MUSEUM

The Big Pit, Blaenafon, is at the north-east corner of the South Wales Coalfield, close to Abergavenny. The colliery was sunk to its present level in 1880, but there are underground shafts and tunnels that date from early as 1812. The coal and iron ore extracted from the mine supplied the famous Blaenafon Ironworks, just a mile away across the Afon Lwyd valley, where modern iron smelting processes were pioneered. In the nineteenth century South Wales' mines helped provide

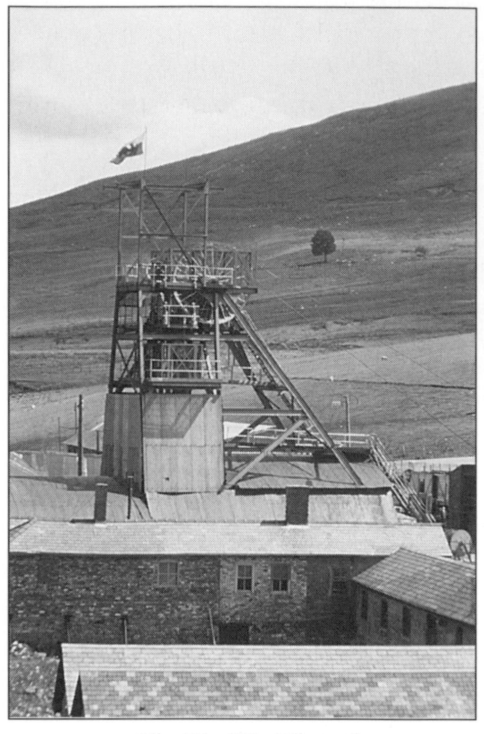

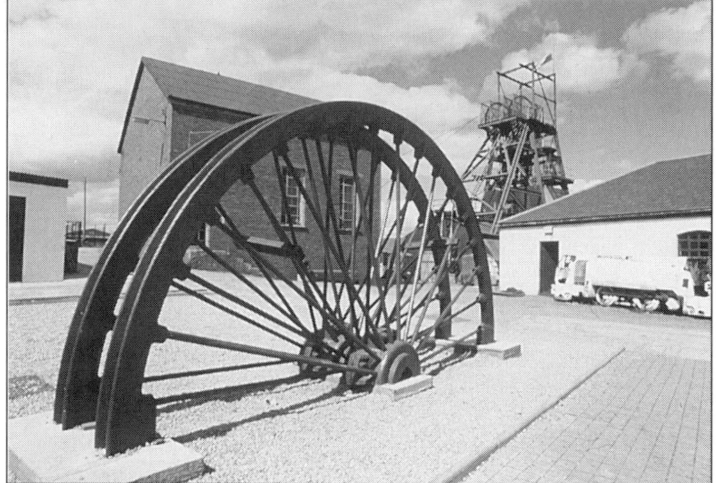

FIGURE 3.1 *The Big Pit, Blaenafon*

the power for the factories, mills, railways and ships of Britain's great period of industrial expansion. Output from the coalfield peaked in 1913 and, at its busiest, the Big Pit employed 1,300 men and boys. Slow decline followed, and by 1966, the Big Pit was the only deep mine left in the Blaenafon area. By 1980, when the last coal was produced, the workforce was a mere 250.

In April 1983, not long after its closure as a working coalmine, the Big Pit (like the Ironworks across the valley) became a museum of South Welsh industrial and social history. The Colliery is now owned by a charitable trust, whose members comprise representatives of local authorities and regional museums. Approximately 50 staff are employed at the site, some on a seasonal basis, and nearly all with personal experience of the mining industry. Since opening, the Big Pit has welcomed over one and a quarter million visitors, and is Britain's most popular coal mining museum, as well as one of Wales' top tourist attractions.

The highlight of a visit to the Big Pit is undoubtedly the underground tour, where groups are taken below the surface to see working conditions for themselves. The guided tours are conducted by experienced miners and last about an hour below ground. Visitors spend about ten minutes being kitted out with helmets, cap lamps, belts, batteries and 'self-rescuers', having 'contraband' collected (see page 21), and riding down the shaft. The 90 metre descent is made by pit cage. In groups of about 17, visitors are taken through underground roadways, air doors, stables and engine houses built by past generations of mineworkers. Back on the surface, the colliery buildings can be explored – the winding engine house, the blacksmith's workshop, the pit-head baths – and more can be learnt about the story of coal from exhibitions and simulated mining galleries. The old miners' canteen is now a comfortable licensed cafeteria with panoramic views of the town of Blaenafon in the valley below. There is a gift shop, well stocked with souvenirs, Welsh crafts and mining memorabilia.

Health, safety and security legislation and the Big Pit

The management of the Big Pit has to take into account not only the health, safety and security legislation that applies to all industry in general, but also the regulations that specifically apply to coal mines. In addition, the manager has introduced voluntary measures, the 'manager's rules and plans'; these are codes of practice directed at health, safety and security hazards relating specifically to this organisation.

The Big Pit closely adheres to all aspects of the Health and Safety at Work Act (1974). Obviously, some of the statutory regulations will have more pertinence to the Big Pit than others. The most important are as follows.

- **The management of health and safety at work regulations (1992)**
  As an operator of a potentially hazardous site, (relative to other tourist attractions) the management of the Big Pit take their obligations seriously under this regulation to assess plan, train and report, in order to ensure all aspects of health and safety are covered for their staff and visitors.
- **Personal protective equipment at work regulations (1992)**
  The underground walkways are dark and the ceilings are low. All staff and visitors are provided with safety helmets and lamps of the type used in working coalmines, as well as personal respirators should air quality deteriorate.
- **Health and safety (safety signs and signals) regulations (1996)**
  Standard signs – for example hard hat areas and no smoking – are clearly displayed on all important routeways.
- **Health and safety (first aid) regulations (1981)**
  There is a carefully planned system of staff training in all aspects of first aid, and adequate equipment is always on hand. The standard kept reflects not only the 1974 Act, but also stricter requirements under the 1954 Mines and Quarries Act (see below) and the first aid in mines regulations.
- **The manual handling operations regulations (1992) and COSHH (1994)** are enforced, as the Big Pit is still regarded by management as an industrial site.
- **The health and safety (display screen equipment) regulations (1992)** have been implemented in the form of improved seating and lighting in the company offices.
- **Reporting of injuries, diseases and dangerous occurrences regulations (1995)**
  Any mishaps on the site are reported, strictly according to the regulations.

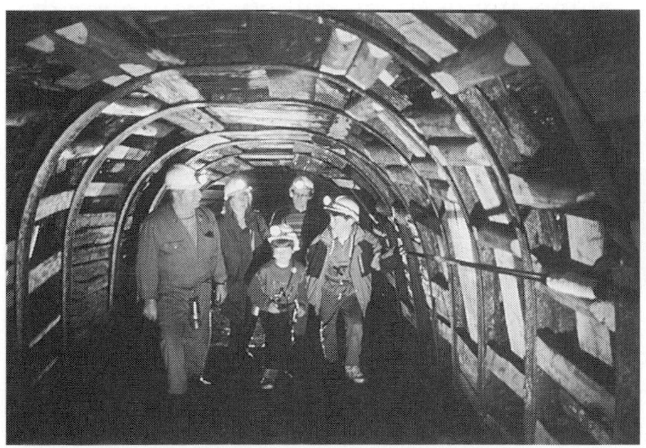

FIGURE 3.2 *All visitors to the Big Pit are provided with personal protective equipment*

The workplace (health, safety and welfare) regulations (1992) do not apply to coal mines, and the provision and use of work equipment regulations (1992) are subservient in the case of the Big Pit to more appropriate laws aimed specifically at mining machinery, under the Mines and Quarries Act (1954). This Act covers safety procedures and maintenance standards at all underground and surface mines and quarries. The manager of every mine must ensure that all equipment is safely installed, commissioned and operated. Furthermore, the manager is required to prepare and keep up to date a suitably written scheme for the systematic inspection, testing, maintenance and (where necessary) repair, renewal or decommissioning of the plant and equipment, under the supervision of qualified, competent and authorised persons. Some of the most important regulations under this Act affecting the Big Pit are:

- the management and administration of safety and health in mines regulations
- shafts and windings regulations
- emergency egress regulations
- the escape from mines regulations
- fire and rescue regulations
- first aid in mines regulations.

The Tips Act (1969) governs the condition of slag heaps and waste tips from a variety of industries, whether the tips are still in use or not.

In addition to the above are the Acts relating to running a catering establishment or shop: the Food Safety Act (1990), the Consumer Protection Act (1987) and the Sale of Goods Act (1979). Finally, as maintenance and customer information is filed on computers, the Data Protection Act (1984) is also important.

The implementation of health, safety and security at the Big Pit

In choosing to take their visitors 90 metres underground into what, despite ostensibly today being a museum and tourist attraction, nevertheless remains a coal mine, the management of the Big Pit have set themselves considerable problems to overcome. All the normal safety procedures that apply to a working coal mine have to be implemented, as well as the added dimensions of caring for visitors unaccustomed to the potential hazards associated with mining.

In reality, visitors to the Big Pit are very safe, for although mining is inherently dangerous, the fact that coal is no longer produced means that the hazards associated with the extractive process (gas, rock falls, contact with machinery) are no longer present, and the chief causes of accidents are immediately eliminated.

The worst case scenario recognised by the management is the breakdown of the winding gear while visitors are in transit in the shaft. Various minor mechanical and electrical problems that could result in such a situation can be dealt with, given a little time, utilising procedures and equipment designed for the purpose. However, a more serious breakdown could require the use of the area's mobile emergency winder, housed at the Big Pit, one of only eight in Britain, and the only one in South Wales. As such a situation could lead to a group of 17 visitors becoming trapped in a crowded pit cage for three or four hours, much responsibility would fall on the shoulders of the guide travelling with them. The Big Pit produces a safety procedures document for guides which includes their duties in such an extreme case.

The 'manager's rules and plans' for health, safety and security at the Big Pit are summarised as follows:

1 The manager of the mine has direct responsibility for health, safety and security.
2 It is the duty of the manager to keep up to date with legislation relating to health, safety and security, and sound operating practices relating specifically to mines via:
    - the Health and Safety Executive mining department
    - the network of colliery managers that exists to collate experience and strategies in this area
    - subscription to Croner's 'Health and Safety in Practice' (see page 36), which collates information on health and safety
    - membership of the Institution of Mining Engineers.
3 Risk assessment leads to the production of written materials which are circulated to employees. At present these are:
    - an Induction Pack for all new employees including, among other things, basic

initial information on health, safety, security and training
- Duties and Procedures for guides (see Figure 3.3): an induction booklet for new tour guides
- maintenance procedures
- COSHH training summaries.

4 The management recognises that training is a vital aspect of maintaining health, safety and security standards. There are three levels of training.

- **Induction**
  Every new member of staff is introduced to the organisation's basic requirements according to current legislation.
- **Statutory qualifications**
  Some of these are essential for mining personnel to carry out their various responsibilities. For instance, the mine manager must by law have a first class certificate of competence as a mining engineer. Some certificates have to be renewed periodically, such as the deputy's gas and hearing certificate, and the first aid at work certificate – these are renewable every three years after courses at Dinas Mines Rescue Station. Non-statutory qualifications for posts which require formal authorisation are assessed internally after in-house training, for instance, for winding enginemen.
- **Health and safety training for specific areas include:**
  - use of oxygen and entenox (one-day course at Dinas)
  - first aid in mines (one-day course at Dinas)
  - safe use of compressed gases (one-day course at British Oxygen Company).

5 The Maintenance policy falls into two broad categories:

- planned preventative maintenance
- curative maintenance after breakdowns.

Obviously, because of the hazards associated with the mining environment, the former is the normal maintenance arrangement. Schedules for inspection and maintenance are observed in accordance to the 1954 Mines and Quarries Act's requirements.

6 The mines inspectors of the Health and Safety Executive visit the Big Pit three or four times every year. They are renowned for their in-depth knowledge of the industry and unswerving adherence to the law. Every effort is made to assist them in their work and to implement their recommendations.

7 Every department of the organisation keeps its own records of health, safety and maintenance activity. These are collated and kept secure within the administration department, which also holds personnel records, financial records, and visitor information. Access to the records is restricted to senior management, except, of course, in cases where the Data Protection Act (1984) applies.

8 Accidents to visitors are prevented by a number of special measures:

- all visitors underground are provided with safety helmets and cap lamps, and 'self-rescuers' (personal respirators for use in emergencies)
- before taking a party underground guides collect and keep under lock and key any 'contraband' – cigarettes, tobacco, matches, lighters, battery operated watches, calculators, radios, personal stereos, cameras – that may create a spark and cause a fire
- groups are kept small for safety reasons. A guide is considered capable of managing a group of around 17 people
- if accompanied by parents, the minimum age at which children are allowed to take the underground tour is five years. For school groups, the minimum age is seven. This is not only because young children need extra supervision, but because the protective clothing is not designed for them.

Statutory Duties

In addition to the specific health and safety duties that individual companies may give their employees, every employee in Britain, regardless of their job or the company they work for, has certain statutory (or legal) duties imposed on them. A detailed copy of the actual regulations in question is available on request but in plain language, they are as follows:

It is the duty of all employees while at work:

- to carry out their duties in accordance with the training and instructions given to them by their employer to ensure compliance with legal requirements;
- to report any dangerous situations in the workplace or any shortcomings in the arrangements for health and safety;
- to take care for the health and safety of themselves and others who may be affected by something they either do or fail to do;
- to co-operate with their employer in his complying with health and safety legislation;
- not to interfere with or misuse anything provided for the purposes of health and safety.

Operational Duties and Procedures for Guides

The following has been drawn up with the help and experience of past and present guides and is designed to ensure that all guides are aware of their duties and the procedures to be adopted in various circumstances to ensure the safety of our visitors, the guides themselves, and the mine.

Responsibility for Visitors

The guide shall be responsible for the safety and welfare of visitors while they are in his charge. That is from the time he takes their contraband from them to the time he returns it or until the party has returned all lamps and helmets.

Contraband

It is the duty of the guide to ensure that all visitors in his party are aware of the rules regarding contraband and to take such contraband from them and lock it in a secure place before taking the party below ground and to return it to them on returning to the surface. If on returning the contraband any visitor claims that their property is missing the guide is to inform the deputy on duty immediately. To reduce the risk of this happening the guide should keep his party together until all contraband items have been returned, so that "missing" items may be checked for immediately. If the guide suspects or is informed that a visitor still has contraband on them during the underground tour then he is to take that contraband from the visitor and retain it in his possession until returning to the surface.

2.3 Intoxication

If before going below ground the guide suspects that a visitor is in a state of intoxication then he is to refuse that visitor entry to the mine and inform the deputy on duty immediately. If he suspects or is informed that a visitor is in an intoxicated state during the underground tour he is to immediately inform the deputy on duty and bring the whole party to the surface.

2.4 Visitor Numbers

It is the duty of the guide to make himself aware of the number of persons in his party before going below ground. The guide shall check on the number of persons in his party as appropriate during the tour and before returning to the surface.

If during the underground tour a guide becomes aware that one of his party is missing he is to make such a search of the immediate vicinity as is practicable without having to leave the rest of his party unattended. If this search is unsuccessful he is to inform the deputy on duty via the nearest tannoy and then wait at that point until the following party arrives. If the missing person or persons are not with the following party the guide is to return the remainder of his party to the surface and then proceed back underground with the deputy to search for the missing person or persons. Any guide who finds any unattended visitor below ground is to immediately inform the deputy on duty and ensure that the person or persons found stay with his party for the rest of the tour or are returned to their proper party.

2.5 Disorderly Behaviour

If at any time during the tour underground a guide finds a member of his party behaving in such a manner which is disruptive or dangerous he shall immediately warn the person that their actions are a danger to others and themselves. The guide shall also warn the person that if their actions continue, the tour will be terminated immediately. If the party is a group booking the guide may appeal for some assistance from the leader of the group at this point.

If the person or persons continue behaving in a disruptive or dangerous manner the guide shall inform the deputy on duty and bring the whole party to the surface immediately. If the persons behaviour is so bad or they refuse to obey the guides instructions he shall inform the deputy on duty and remain at that point with his party until another member of staff arrives to assist him.

If the party is made up of casual visitors and the tour has in any way been disrupted by the behaviour of any person then the guide shall apologise on behalf of the museum and if necessary offer the party the chance of another tour of the mine.

2.6 Accident

If during the underground tour any visitor is injured or becomes unwell the guide shall:

- If it is a minor injury not requiring immediate treatment, inform the visitor that they will be treated on arrival at the surface.
- If it is a minor injury requiring immediate treatment either give such treatment (from one of the first aid boxes) or inform the deputy on duty, who will come and give treatment.

- If it is a more serious injury (i.e. broken bone, unconsciousness, severe bleeding etc.) inform the deputy on duty immediately and give such treatment as possible.

2.7 Finding Something Dangerous

If at any time on the underground tour the guide finds anything of a dangerous nature e.g. broken timbers, small falls etc. he shall assess whether it is safe for his party to pass. If he considers it safe he may proceed with his party but must inform the deputy of the nature and extent of the problem.

If the guide considers it unsafe to pass he must return via the the route he has come informing the deputy and the guides of the following parties of the nature and extent of the problem.

Any party who's tour has been seriously disrupted shall be offered another of the unaffected side of the mine.

2.8 Fire

If at any time during the underground tour a guide detects any indication of fire (e.g. smell or sight of) he shall immediately inform the deputy on duty of the nature and extent of the indication. The Deputy having investigated will then decide whether it is safe for the tour to continue or whether it is necessary to evacuate the mine. If the guide sees any indication of open fire he is to immediately inform the deputy on duty and return to the surface via the route indicated by the Deputy.

2.9 Emergency Egress

2.9.1 From the Shaft

If at any time the cage stops in the shaft for a period exceeding **5** minutes the following sequence of events will take place:

(i) **Communication** - The Mine Deputy or Banksman will contact the guide via the surface-to-cage intercomm *(all guides will have been given instruction on how to operate these)* and inform him of the nature of the breakdown i.e. Mechanical or Electrical.

(ii) **Use of the Emergency Generator** - If the fault cannot be rectified within a reasonable amount of time then the procedure for operating the Emergency Generator will be carried out by the engineering staff. This procedure could take up to 30 mins to complete and involves the use of the generator to produce enough electricity to release the winder brakes. This in turn will allow the winding cycle to be completed by gravity and then allow the guide to escort his party out of the mine via River Arch *(see below)*.

(iii) **Use of the Mobile Winder** - In the event of a major mechanical breakdown where the emergency generator would not be of use or if the cages became physically stuck in the shaft i.e. by a guide rope breaking or ravelling, then the Mobile Winder would have to be called out.
At present the Mobile Winder is garaged at Big Pit but ***all guides should note that it is likely to take about 3½ hours to set up the winder and begin raising persons to the surface.***
If the circumstances were to occur which necessitated the use of the Mobile Winder then the guides' role will obviously be the most vital and difficult of all those inviolved.
The guides' first task is to calmly reassure the visitors of their safety. **"THEY ARE SAFE, IT WILL JUST TAKE TIME TO GET THEM OUT"**. Next, the guide should explain the sequence of events and the procedure that is about to take place. So, it is important that the guide fully understands the procedure himself. (A detailed description of the Mobile Winder procedure is available from the Mechanical Engineer). As the visitors are going to have to remain in the cage for 4 hours or more they will need to be made as comfortable as possible and it may be necessary for some of them to remove their lamps if they become too uncomfortable.

(iv) **Via River Arch** - Circumstances may arise which will require the Deputy to issue instructions for the evacuation of the mine via the River Arch. On being instructed to exit via River Arch by the Deputy, the guide will inform the Deputy of the location and number of visitors in his party and whether he will require assistance with anyone in his party because of their age or infirmity. Any visitors in wheelchairs should be placed in the charge of the Hitcher as special arrangements involving extra personnel will be necessary to evacuate them. Before setting off for River Arch the guide is to inform the surface of the time he is setting off and the number of visitors in his party. The first guide to start off will take the key for the River Arch gate from its position and inform the surface that he has done so. Guides are reminded that it is quite a long walk to the exit from River Arch and so they should make frequent stops for the visitors to rest on the way out. At the exit they will be met by other members of staff with whatever transport is available to take them back to the museum. In the vast majority of cases in which this procedure is put into use the reason for doing so will be because of a problem with the Winder rather than because of any danger underground. The guide should therefore reassure the visitors of their safety at all times and try to make the whole procedure seem like an extended tour rather than an emergency evacuation.

3. Conclusion

The above are your duties and you will be expected to be fully familiar with the contents of this document, but as was stated at the beginning, it has been drawn up using the experience and knowledge of our present guides. In the hope that we learn something every day, however, please don't hesitate to suggest any improvements or additions or to make any other comment on the above as it has been drawn up for your benefit and for that of your successors.

SOURCE: *The Big Pit*
FIGURE 3.3 *The Big Pit's induction booklet for new tour guides*

- disorderly or disruptive behaviour by visitors will not be tolerated
- there are numerous signs both underground and on the surface warning visitors of safe practice. Fire fighting equipment is visible throughout the tour
- to prevent trips and falls, the ground surface of the mine has been greatly improved.

Conclusions

The Big Pit practices exemplary standards of health, safety and security, and exceeds the requirements of the law with its own voluntary codes of practice. It hardly needs to be pointed out that a tourist attraction of this nature could be potentially very hazardous, if standards were allowed to lapse. The efforts made by the management and staff of the Big Pit ensure its survival not only as a stimulating museum, but also as a much needed source of employment and income in post-industrial Blaenafon.

THORPE PARK

Thorpe Park is one of Britain's leading family leisure parks, occupying a 500 acre site in Surrey, close to the M25. It is owned and operated by a subsidiary of RMC (Ready-Mixed Concrete Group Plc), who had the foresight to develop the ex-gravel pit for leisure use. With over half the area consisting of lakes, Thorpe Park maintains its original aquatic theme, while millions of pounds have been invested on new rides and attractions since it opened in 1979.

Thorpe Park is a substantial organisation and employs a large number of people, not only to operate the rides, but also to develop and landscape the site and carry out maintenance, cleaning, catering, retailing, marketing, administration and security. With such a large staff, and with over a million visitors a year enjoying Thorpe Park's attractions, it is self-evident that issues of health, safety and security occupy a large part of its management's time.

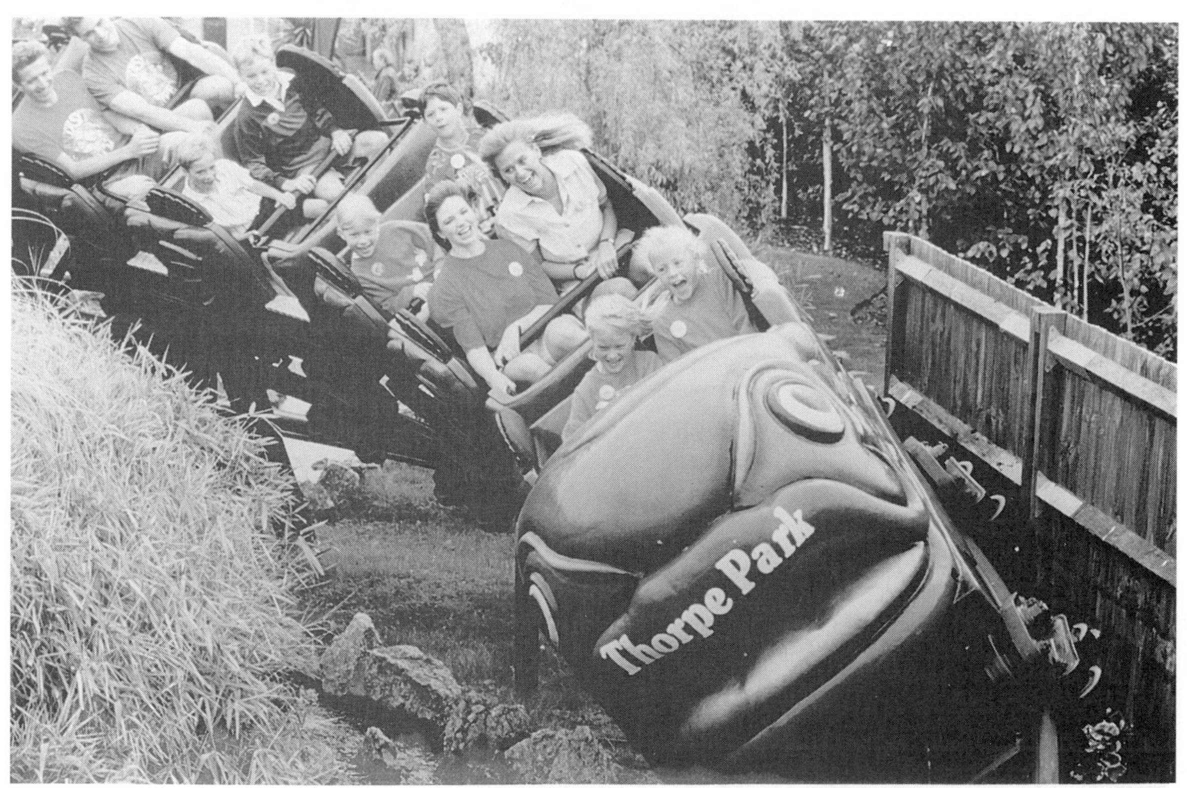

SOURCE: *Thorpe Park*
FIGURE 3.4 *Every ride at Thorpe Park is inspected daily*

Health, safety and security legislation and Thorpe Park

The scale of Thorpe Park's operations means that none of the regulations under the Health and Safety at Work Act (1974) are without relevance. However, the necessity to cope with thousands of people at any one time throws stress on particular areas. For instance, the health and safety (safety signs and signals) regulations (1996) are rigorously enforced to inform visitors of safety procedures and exit routes in enclosed areas, in order to ensure rapid evacuation in the case of fire. The local authority and fire brigade are intimately involved with the lay-out of new attractions, and the provision of fire-fighting equipment.

With so many people to cater for, the health and safety (first aid) regulations (1981) require Thorpe Park to provide a comprehensive service. In fact, the park has a fully equipped first aid centre, with two nurses, rescue 'buggies' driven by trained first-aiders, and its own ambulance. In all, over 50 of the staff have either basic or advanced first aid training, and can give assistance in any emergency from a grazed knee to a heart attack. The first aid centre is marked on a map of the park which is given to all visitors on arrival. If accidents occur, RMC has its own internal system of written reports, in addition to the statutory requirements under RIDDOR (1995).

With a large catering and retail side to its operation, Thorpe Park pays close attention to the Consumer Protection Act (1987), the Sale of Goods Act (1979) and the Food Safety Act (1990). Because a computer filing system is used for staff and customer records, the Data Protection Act (1984) also applies.

Although no statutory regulation or other Act applies specifically to fairgrounds and theme parks, the Health and Safety Executive publish a series of codes of practice for the operation of individual types of rides, as well as an overall summary of good procedure – 'Fairgrounds and amusement parks: a code of safe practice' (1992). Every aspect of designing, installing and operating a ride, its maintenance and the training of staff, are covered by the code, which is strictly enforced by the management.

Finally, from its opening, the nature of the site, with its many deep water lakes, has lent Thorpe Park an aquatic character. 'Thorpe Farm' is reached by waterbuses across one of the lakes. Under Section 85 of the Merchant Shipping Act (1995), the waterbuses must be operated by a person qualified with a boat master's licence, and be regularly inspected by the Marine Safety Agency.

The implementation of health, safety and security at Thorpe Park

The management of Thorpe Park is acutely aware of the hazards posed by a combination of rides, water and young children, and have gone to great lengths to ensure the safety of all their visitors. The ultimate responsibility for health and safety is assumed by the parent company (RMC) in their statement of company policy (see Figure 3.5).

All new employees are issued with an induction booklet which dedicates a large section to their role in health and safety matters, and this is reinforced during their basic training. RMC has its own safety department, and liaises with Thorpe Park's own safety manager during regular meetings.

Thorpe Park works closely with the HSE, especially during the planning stage of new rides, and are responsible for considerable input. However, during the day-to-day operation of the park, the local authority and fire brigade have more involvement through routine inspections and advice on safe practice.

The management keeps up to date on health and safety issues through subscription to Croner's 'Health and Safety in Practice', its subscription to *Health and Safety in Europe* (the journal of the British Safety Industry Federation), and through its membership of

RMC Health & Safety Policy in the U.K.

Statement

As Executive Director of the RMC Group of Companies, with overall responsibility for the Group's operations in the Retail, Merchanting & Leisure Divisions, I wish to emphasise my commitment to the achievement and maintenance of high standards of health and safety.

The management of health and safety is an integral part of the Group's management responsibilities. The U.K. Health & Safety Council, of which I am Joint Chairman, is responsible to the Main Board for health and safety matters in the U.K. It is the duty of management at all levels to ensure that the organisation and arrangements for health and safety are clearly laid down, constantly reviewed, and effectively implemented.

Organisation

Divisional Managing Directors, with Divisional Directors and Managers, and others with senior management jurisdiction, are required to ensure that effective health and safety policies are implemented, and to set out health and safety objectives which will support the achievement of high standards.

General Managers are required to establish that effective health and safety arrangements are applied to the day to day management of their companies in line with divisional requirements.

Arrangements

Management, at all levels, are responsible for the implementation of the following health and safety arrangements:

Planning - that formal health and safety planning and budgeting occurs.

Co-operation and Communication - that systems are established so that health and safety issues are freely discussed, and that information is communicated to employees and third parties, and shared with other Group companies.

Competence - that sufficient quality health and safety training is provided for all employees.

Monitoring and Review - that regular health and safety inspections and audits are undertaken and that systems are reviewed in the light of their findings.

The U.K. Health & Safety Department, and Divisional Health & Safety Managers, are responsible for providing a quality service to support the effective management of health and safety.

It is the objective of the RMC Group in the U.K. that, by proper organisation and implementation of formal arrangements, all managers and employees remain constantly aware of health and safety hazards, and take rapid and effective measures to minimise any associated risks.

July 1996 Signed ....

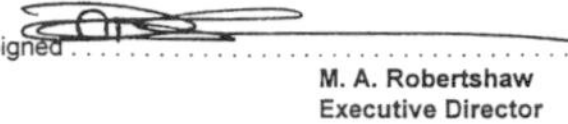

M. A. Robertshaw
Executive Director

FIGURE 3.5 *RMC's statement of company policy for new tour guides*

BALPPA (the British Association of Leisure Parks, Piers and Attractions). This organisation has a safety committee which notifies its members of relevant changes in legislation and acts in an advisory capacity. Training is considered a high priority at Thorpe Park, and staff participate regularly in courses such as fire fighting, first aid and those of NEBOSH (the national examination board in occupational safety and health).

As well as employing the duty manager, one of whose daily responsibilities is to walk through the park looking out for potential hazards, Thorpe Park operates an effective and rigorous system of maintenance on its rides. Written risk assessments are produced by ride managers and, if necessary, external agencies are called in to advise. On a daily basis, all rides are inspected by mechanics and electricians at 7.30 am and by a system of cards (green for mechanical, white for electrical) the operators are informed that the ride is safe to use. If a red card is left on the ride, it means that there is a problem, the ride will not be opened, and visitors will be informed of this at the gate. At the end of each season, the rides are completely dismantled and overhauled.

The sheer number of visitors in mid-season at Thorpe Park presents its own particular security problems. In the case of fire, the rapid movement of large numbers of people will need to be monitored and coordinated. To this end, the park has a closed circuit television system (CCTV) feeding into a central control room – 'Thorpe Control'. A fire alarm panel informs the controller of the precise location of any emergency, and he or she is in contact with no less than 70 staff who are equipped with two-way radios. The CCTV system also has obvious advantages in protecting the public from the attention of pickpockets, or other criminals that may be attracted by the crowds.

Finally, some measure of Thorpe Park's dedication to the welfare of their visitors may be gained by their recent practice exercise, in which a mock train collision was staged on the 'Canada Creek Railway'. The emergency services participated in the treatment and evacuation of a number of 'casualties', and much was learned that has contributed to health and safety planning for the future.

Conclusion

Thorpe Park is a major leisure venue on a national scale, and a family seeking to enjoy the excitement of its rides would be justified in expecting only the most dedicated commitment to their safety from its staff. Clearly, they would not be disappointed by our brief look behind the scenes. The presence of water, large numbers of people, and the 'state-of-the-art' rides themselves all pose particular problems for Thorpe Park's management, and we have learned how these are overcome by the management's own careful planning and implementation of the safety procedures required by law.

SECTION

4

The Tasks

The three tasks contained in this section ask you to develop and demonstrate your understanding of health, safety and security issues.

As future employees of the leisure and tourism industries, it is important for you to understand, and be able to put into practice, key laws and regulations relating to health, safety and security. You should investigate how health, safety and security applies to leisure and tourism organisations. You must establish which laws apply to each organisation and the measures taken to comply with the law. You may wish to use one (or both) of the two case studies in the previous section as material for your evidence, or as examples of the kind of study you can produce on your own. At some stage you will need to visit your own chosen organisation(s) to interview the manager in charge of health, safety and security to collection information for your case study. In order to give a structure to the interview, you may wish to design a questionnaire similar to that illustrated in Figure 4.1.

THE RELEVANCE OF KEY LAWS AND REGULATIONS TO ORGANISATIONS

ORGANISATION: ____________________

NAME OF PERSON INTERVIEWED: ____________________

Which of the following Laws and Regulations mostly apply to you? Could you select the ones that have most relevance to your organisation and give an example how you comply with this legislation.

1. The Health and Safety at Work Act (1974)

   * The Management of Health and Safety at Work Regulations (1992)
   * The Workplace (Health, Safety and Welfare) Regulations (1992)
   * Personal Protective Equipment at Work Regulations (1992)
   * Manual Handling Operations Regulations (1992)
   * Provision and Use of Work Equipment Regulations (1992)
   * Health and Safety (Display Screen Equipment) Regulations (1992)
   * The Control of Substances Hazardous to Health Regulations (1994)
   * Health and Safety (Safety Signs and Signals) Regulations (1996)
   * Reporting of Injuries, Diseases and Dangerous Occurrences Regulations (1995)
   * Health and Safety (First Aid) Regulations (1981)
   * Noise at Work Regulations (1989)

2. The Food Safety Act (1990)
3. The Fire Precautions Act (1971)
4. Consumer Protection Act (1987)
5. Sale of Goods Act (1979)
6. Data Protection Act (1984)
7. Any others?

QUESTIONS ON HEALTH, SAFETY AND SECURITY TO ASK ON A VISIT TO AN ORGANISATION

1. Could you give me a brief background to your organisation?

2. Which acts, regulations or codes of practice apply to your organisation? (use accompanying form)

3. What measures do you take to ensure that your organisation complies with health, safety and security legislation?

4. Could you give me an example of a health, safety or security hazard faced by your organisation and how you dealt with it?

FIGURE 4.1 *A suggested questionnaire for a management interview on health, safety and security*

TASK 1

You are required to prepare a wordprocessed report explaining the relevance of key laws and regulations on health, safety and security in relation to four leisure and tourism organisations, two from leisure and recreation and two from travel and tourism. Provide brief backgrounds to the organisations to set the scene. Take a general approach at first, aquainting yourself with all Acts and regulations that apply to the chosen businesses and include these in your report.

After this explanation, concentrate on the legislation that has particular relevance to the businesses in question. Make sure that you include not only the Acts, regulations and codes of practice that are applicable to all businesses, but also those that are specific to the nature of the organisation you are describing.

Complete your report by indicating the measures taken by the organisations to ensure they comply with health, safety and security legislation.

CHECKLIST OF PORTFOLIO EVIDENCE

- ☑ Wordprocessed report on four organisations.
- ☑ Completed questionnaire.

TASK 2

For Task 1 you explained the relevance of key laws and regulations in relation to four leisure and tourism organisations. You are now required to select one of these organisations in order to write an induction booklet (for an example see Figure 3.3) on health, safety and security for a trainee manager of this facility.

The induction booklet needs to explain clearly to the new member of staff, practices and procedures used by the organisation to ensure the health, safety and security of employees and visitors, and the legislation with which it has to comply. The booklet should be designed in five sections to explain:

1 Why it is important for the organisation to maintain high levels of care in health, safety and security. This section could be an introduction to the booklet.
2 The measures undertaken by the organisation to ensure that they comply with health, safety and security legislation. This section should focus on how the organisation implements the demands of the law, e.g. warning signs, training and first aid. It should describe both obligatory and voluntary measures.
3 An explanation of the purposes of laws and regulations. This section should give the trainee an insight into the value of health, safety and security legislation in order to encourage him or her to enforce the legal requirements.
4 The sources of information about key laws and regulations. The trainee should have guidance on where to go to seek further professional advice on health, safety and security.
5 The relevance of key laws and regulations to the organisation. This section must indicate all Acts, regulations and codes of practice that apply. It must also list both employer's and employee's responsibilities.

Wordprocess the booklet and, using clip art, include illustrations to make this an appealing and accessible document.

CHECKLIST OF PORTFOLIO EVIDENCE

☑ Wordprocessed induction booklet on health, safety and security

Key Skills Hint: Communication

Task 3 asks you to organise formal meetings and prepare agendas and minutes. Since members of the team need to prepare for a meeting, it is important that they have some idea of the matters to be discussed and the order in which various items will be handled. Your agenda might look like this:

NEWTOWN SIXTH FORM COLLEGE
Leisure event management committee
Meeting to be held in Room 22B, 4 November 1996
AGENDA

1 Apologies for absence
2 Minutes of meeting held 26 October 1966
3 Matters arising from minutes

Items for discussion:

4 Report from Fire Safety sub-group
5 Report from Security sub-group
6 Statement by event treasurer
7 Report by chairperson on response to call for volunteer stewards
8 Any other business
9 Date of next meeting

During the meeting, the secretary will need to ensure that a record of the proceedings is taken down. These will be written up after the meeting and will form the minutes.

The minutes should follow the same order as the agenda and must be an accurate record of what was said and agreed. They need to be written down in concise note form, not word-for-word.

If you are responsible for taking down the minutes at a meeting, the following guidelines should help to ensure that your notes are accurate and relevant.

- Record the date, time and place of the meeting
- Make a list of all the members attending, 'officials' first, and then an alphabetical list of others
- Make a list of apologies for absence, and note reasons given
- Using the agenda as your guide, give each topic a clear sub-heading and briefly summarise the discussion
- Do not attempt to take notes of every word spoken. You need a *summary* of the main facts and arguments
- Ensure that you have statements attributed to the right person. Always note action to be taken by individual members
- Never write your notes from a personal point of view; you need an objective record
- If you are uncertain about any points to be recorded, ask the chairperson at the time and do not leave it until later. If necessary, ask members to wait until you have had time to note important points
- Once you leave the meeting, try to write up the formal minutes as soon as possible
- Make maximum use of layout in your notes and minutes, using capitals, headings, spacings and indentation. Use a referencing system of numbers or letters to identify clearly headings, sub-headings and points
- The minutes should be circulated to the members who attended, absent members and anyone who is required to take some form of action

TASK 3

You are required to act as a member of a team that is ensuring the health, safety and security of an event of your own choosing. This exercise may be combined with your work for the *Event Management* unit. You will need to take part in meetings to:

- decide on the event. In order to achieve the enforcement of realistic measures to ensure health, safety and security, take into account the skills and availability of people involved, as well as finance, time and materials at your disposal
- assess all existing and potential hazards related to the event and evaluate the levels of risk involved
- propose measures for ensuring the health, safety and security of the event, discussing possible ways to reduce risks. Also take into account emergency action should problems occur. Ensure proposals are consistent with legal, regulatory and insurance requirements
- decide on the appropriate sources of expert help, information and advice you intend to consult.

During the meetings, roles should be allocated to each member of the team to share the health, safety and security responsibilities (e.g. contacting the fire authority, researching relevant legislation and the secure handling of money). Some of these roles will require team members to carry out duties prior to the event. Everyone should be involved in these as well as in duties during the event. You are each required to write the minutes of the meetings.

During the event, you will be observed carrying out your role and a record of observation (see Figure 4.2) will be issued to you, evaluating your performance.

CHECKLIST OF PORTFOLIO EVIDENCE

- ☑ Minutes of meetings
- ☑ Record of Observation
- ☑ Detailed notes made by you to prepare for meetings, and in undertaking your event

FURTHER SOURCES OF INFORMATION ABOUT HEALTH, SAFETY AND SECURITY

The completion of Task 3 will require some research on your part. There are many sources of information on health, safety and security, and even for experts it is a full time job to keep up to date. To help you, this section has been prepared to give some initial

Key Skills Hint

Depending on the event chosen, many key skills may be claimed for Task 3. For example, a health and fitness exhibition held within a hall could include the following exercise:

'Estimate the size of the hall, measure it, draw a plan of the area, and on paper cut to size, overlay the stands, tables and equipment, that will be used so that you can decide on the layout of the exhibition.'

All performance criteria from application of number can be evidenced by this task. This, however, only covers part of the evidence indicators and all performance criteria will have to be covered again in order to meet the full requirements of the application of number unit.

HEALTH, SAFETY AND SECURITY IN LEISURE AND TOURISM
RECORD OF OBSERVATION

NAME OF STUDENT: ______________________________

NAME OF ASSESSOR: ______________________________

The above named student took part in ensuring the health, safety and security of the following event: ______________________________

____

on: ______________________________

as part of the requirements of the Advanced GNVQ in Leisure and Tourism.

Comments on student's performance: ______________________________

____

____

____

____

____

____

____

Requirements of Evidence Indicator Met: _______ Not Met: _______

Signature of Student : ______________________________

Signature of Assessor: ______________________________

Date: ______________

FIGURE 4.2 *Suggested record of observation*

guidance into this vast area of expertise. Hopefully, it will be of use not only for the purposes of Task 3, but also in your subsequent employment in the leisure and tourism industry.

If you want to study the actual terminology of the Health and Safety at Work Act (1974), or any of the other Acts of Parliament mentioned in this book, you can find them in full in *Halsbury's Statutes of England And Wales*, (Butterworths, London). Similarly, the statutory regulations are to be found in *Halsbury's Statutory Instruments* (Butterworths, London). You should be able to find copies of these at a good local reference library. Individual copies of the legislation are available from HMSO.

However, it is rarely necessary, or of benefit for those without a legal background to wade through the sometimes convoluted language of these legal texts. In most instances, the primary source of information and advice about health and safety at work in Great Britain are the publications of the Health and Safety Executive. The central office of the HSE is in London, but the contact point for public enquiries is: the health and safety infoline (01541 545500). There are about 40 area offices of the HSE, and their numbers can be found in your local telephone directory. In addition, the HSE maintains an autofax service on 01839 060606, and the British Library has a database of over 150,000 publications on health and safety at work. In Northern Ireland, the contact address is:

The Health and Safety Agency for Northern Ireland, 83, Ladas Drive, Belfast BT6 9FJ. (01232 243249)

As well as codes of practice and guidance notes to specific regulations, the HSE publishes a wide range of bulletins, newsletters, manuals and reports, many of which are relevant to workplace situations in leisure and tourism. The list below is not exhaustive, but gives an idea of the kind of help available, should you decide to organise an event. These publications are available direct from the HSE, but many of them are expensive. Again, your local reference library should have copies, or your school or college library might obtain them for you. The Health and Safety Agency for Northern Ireland publish their own series of codes of practice and guidance notes, many closely modelled on the British equivalents.

The following list gives details of some of the HSE publications of most interest to the leisure and tourism industries.

General information about health and safety at work

- *Current List of Health and Safety Legislation*, 1955, **ISBN 0 7176 1067 5**, £10.50
- *Essentials of Health and Safety at Work* (guidance notes), 1994, **ISBN 0 7176 0716 X**, £5.95
- *A Guide to the Health and Safety at Work Act* (guidance notes), 5th edn, 1992, **ISBN 0 7176 0441 1**, £4.00
- *Workplace Health and Safety in Europe*, 1991, **ISBN 0 11 885614 6**, £9.00
- *Regulation of Health and Safety in Denmark, France, Germany, Spain and Italy* (research report), 1995, **ISBN 0 7176 1013 6**, £60.00
- *The Health and Safety System in Great Britain*, 1992, **ISBN 0 7176 0892 1**, £6.50

The following publications will be of help in implementing other specific statutory regulations.

Workplace requirements

- *Slips and Trips, Guidance for Employers on Identifying Hazards and Controlling Risks* (guidance notes), 1966, **ISBN 0 7176 1145 0**, £7.50
- *Workplace Health, Safety and Welfare Regulations* (code of practice), 1992, **ISBN 0 7176 0413 6**, £5.00
- *Seating At Work* (guidance notes), 1991, **ISBN 0 11 885431 3**, £2.25
- *A Pain in Your Workplace: ergonomic problems and solutions* (guidance notes), 1994, **ISBN 0 7176 0668**, £10.95

Health and safety management

- *Management of Health and Safety at Work Regulations* (code of practice), 1992, **ISBN 7176 0412 8**, £5.00

- *Writing Your Health and Safety Policy Statement: a guide to preparing a safety policy statement for a small business* (guidance notes), 1989, ISBN 0 7176 0424 1, £3.00
- *Health Risk Management: a practical guide for managers in small and medium sized enterprises* (guidance notes), 1995, ISBN 0 7176 0905 7, £6.50
- *You Can Do It. The What, Why and How of Improving Health and Safety at Work*, 1994, ISBN 0 7176 0726 7, £14.50
- *Improving Compliance With Safety Procedures*, 1996, ISBN 0 7176 0970 7, £20.00
- *New and Expectant Mothers at Work: a guide for employers* (guidance notes), 1995, ISBN 0 7176 0826 3, £6.25
- *Violence to Staff: a basis for assessment and prevention*, 1986, ISBN 0 11 883887 3, £3.50

Equipment and manual handling

- *Work Equipment: provision and use of work equipment regulations* (guidance notes), 1992, ISBN 0 7176 0414 4, £5.00
- *Manual Handling: manual handling operations' regulations* (guidance notes), 1992, ISBN 0 7176 0411 x, £5.00
- *Manual Handling – Solutions You Can Handle* (guidance notes), 1994, ISBN 0 7176 06937, £7.95

Personal protective equipment and display screens

- *Personal Protective Equipment at Work* (guidance notes), 1992, ISBN 0 7176 0415 2, £5.00
- *Display Screen Equipment at Work: Health and Safety (Display Screen Equipment) Regulations* (guidance notes), 1992, ISBN 0 7176 0410 9, £5.00

First aid, RIDDOR and warning signs

- *First Aid at Work. Health and Safety (First Aid) Regulations* (code of practice), 1981, ISBN 0 7176 04268, £3.00
- *Safety Signs and Signals* (guidance notes), 1996, ISBN 0 7176 0870 0, £8.50
- *A Guide to RIDDOR* (guidance notes), 1995, ISBN 0 7176 1012 8, £6.95
- *Everyone's Guide to RIDDOR '95* 1995, ISBN 0 7176 1077 2, (single copies free on request)

Care of substances hazardous to health

- *A Step by Step Guide to COSHH Assessment* (guidance notes), 1993, ISBN 0 11 886379 7, £7.00
- *General COSHH, Carcinogens and Biological Agents Regulations* (code of practice), 1995, ISBN 0 7176 0819 0, £6.75

Some HSE publications with special relevance to leisure and tourism situations

- *Managing Crowd Safety in Public Venues: a study to generate guidance for venue owners and enforcing authority inspectors* (research report), 1993, ISBN 0 7176 0708 9, £60.00
- *Zoos: safety, health and welfare standards for employers and persons at work* (code of practice), 1985, ISBN 0 11 883823 7, £3.50
- *Electrical Safety at Places of Entertainment* (guidance notes), 1991, ISBN 0 11 885598 0, £2.50
- *Health and Safety in Horse Riding Establishments* (guidance notes), 1993, ISBN 0 7176 0632 5, £8.50
- *Safety at Outdoor Activity Centres*, 1995, ISBN 0 7176 0822 0, £5.00
- *A Guide to Health, Safety and Welfare at Pop Concerts and Similar Events*, 1993, (published by the Health and Safety Commission, the Home Office and the Scottish Office) ISBN 011 341072 7, £10.00

There is a whole series of publications covering individual fairground rides, but as many events feature the provision of a 'bouncy castle', perhaps you should be aware of:

- *Safe Operation of Passenger Carrying Amusement Devices – Inflatable Bouncing Devices* (guidance notes), 1991, **ISBN 0 11 885604 9**, £2.50
- *Fairgrounds and Amusement Parks: a code of safe practice*, 1992, **ISBN 0 7176 0550**, £4.50

If you are considering a firework display:

- *Working Together on Firework Displays: a guide to safety for firework display organisers and operators* (guidance notes), 1995, **ISBN 0 7176 0835 2**, £8.95

Many leisure events, like discos and concerts, can be noisy:

- *Noise at Work. Noise Assessment, Information and Control* (guidance notes), 1990, **ISBN 0 11 885430 5**, £3.00
- *Sound Solutions: techniques to reduce noise at work*, 1996, **ISBN 0 7176 0791 7**, £10.95

Finally, there are some publications useful for schools and colleges:

- *Health and Safety Management in Higher and Further Education: guidance on inspection, monitoring and auditing*, 1992, **ISBN 0 11 886315 0**, £3.00
- *Audiovisual Resources in Occupational Health and Safety: films, videos and tape slides available from distributors in the United Kingdom* (bibliography), **ISBN 0 7176 0960 X**, £15.00
- *COSHH: guidance for schools* (guidance notes), 1989, **ISBN 0 11 885511 5**, £2.00
- *COSHH: guidance for universities, polytechnics and colleges of further education* (guidance notes), 1990, **ISBN 0 11 885433 X**, £2.00

Other sources

Apart from the Health and Safety Executive, and the Northern Ireland Health and Safety Agency, there are many other sources of advice and information.

- **Your local fire authority** will advise on the provision and choice of any necessary fire-fighting equipment, emergency access and exits, etc
- **The local authority's Environmental Health Department** will have expert knowledge of COSHH, noise hazards, RIDDOR and food hygiene. In fact, local authorities tend to become more involved in the day-to-day running of leisure and tourism venues than the HSE
- **Croner the publisher** produce a continuously updated loose-leaf 'encyclopaedia' of health and safety legislation. There are about 25,000 current subscriptions to this useful source of up-to-date information. Croner can be contacted at Croner House, London Road, Kingston-upon-Thames, Surrey, KT2 6SR (Tel: 0181 5472647)
- **The British Safety Industry Federation** produces a bi-monthly magazine called *Health & Safety Europe*. It is available from BPL Business Publications Ltd, Brooklyn House, 22, The Green, West Drayton, Middlesex, UB7 7PQ (Tel: 01895 421111)
- **The British Safety Council** is an independent campaigning and educational body with the objective of preventing accidents, injury and disease, and promoting health in the workplace. The council promotes health, safety and environmental awareness and helps workplaces to identify and manage risks. The British Safety Council is at the National Safety Centre, 70, Chancellors Road, London W6 9RS
- **Approved courses** on health and safety skills at colleges and education centres throughout the UK are organised by the National Examination Board in Occupational Safety and Health (NEBOSH). They can be contacted at NEBOSH House, The Grange, Highfield Drive, Wigston, Leicester, LE18 1PP (Tel: 0116 2888858)
- **Many commercial companies** today exist to advise on health and safety problems. You may be interested to look up their advertisements listed in Yellow Pages. The HSE will offer their recommendations on the choice of professional consultancy if requested

- Advice on security is always available from the **crime prevention unit** at your local police station
- **The local authority trading standards officer** is the first point of enquiry for help on consumer law. More serious problems may be referred to the Department of Trade and Industry
- **The Data Protection Registrar** is located at Wycliffe House, Water Lane, Wilmslow, Cheshire, SK9 5AF (Tel: 01625 545745)
- **Other organisations**, such as the Sports Council and the Royal Society for the Prevention of Accidents may be able to offer advice. Finally, don't hesitate to ask for some tips from any local organisations or charities that regularly run fund-raising events: they may come up with some useful ideas, as long as you don't ring at a busy time!

SECTION

5

Review of Unit

Key Aims

Working through this section you will:

- briefly review areas studied in Sections 1–4
- consider the effect of recently published guidance, on the organisation of public events
- complete a task designed to help you consider the wider implications of health, safety and security legislation

So far, you have:

- studied key laws and regulations for health, safety and security in Great Britain and Northern Ireland
- learnt how these laws apply to selected leisure and tourism organisations
- produced written health, safety and security guidance for new employees of an organisation
- ensured the health, safety and security of your own event.

Not everyone is happy with the way legislation seems to impinge more and more on individual liberties. Some may think that the law has already gone far enough. For instance, there must be countless miles of unused shelving in the UK, now deemed either too high or too low by wary employers, but previously used for years without problems. A few people living within earshot of motor racing circuits, in houses built long after the tracks were first used, can use new environmental legislation to put an end to the sport thousands come to enjoy. The best-intentioned legislation can result in stifling over-protection, or can protect one person while denying the liberty of another. To end the unit, it may be appropriate to consider a situation which at this moment is causing great concern to event managers across Europe.

THE INSTITUTE OF STRUCTURAL ENGINEERS' REPORT (1995)

At the end of 1995, the Institute of Structural Engineers (ISE) produced their controversial publication, *Temporary Demountable Structures – Guidance on Procurement, Design and Use.* This came about as a result of the collapse, with great loss of life, of a seating grandstand at Bastia in Corsica in May 1992. The guidance covers not only seating structures but also temporary stages, of the type used at music festivals and outdoor concerts.

However, events organisers are dismayed because they feel that very few of them will be able to comply with the ISE guidelines. It is required that chartered engineers are involved throughout the process of design, hire and use of temporary structures used at events. An engineer would need to design or advise on the hiring of a stage, check documentation, liaise with local authorities and supervise the construction process. Event organisers fear this would mean the end of thousands of events, where compliance to these demands would be beyond the financial constraints of the organisers. Besides, it is doubted if there are even enough chartered engineers in the UK to do this extra work. Associations of events organisers and allied corporations are upset by the ISE's lack of consultation before producing their guidelines, and claim that the document contradicts existing HSE guidance. Although the ISE publication carries no legal force as such, an event organiser who disregarded it could be in serious trouble in a civil action in court at a later date, should an accident occur. Also, some local authorities, who have the power to refuse licenses, are already insisting on compliance to ISE procedures, presumably with a mind to their own legal position.

The Events Services Association and the Production Services Association have produced their own document in response, asking for the ISE guidelines to be withdrawn. They feel the ISE was naive to publish them with apparently little idea of the turmoil they would cause in the world of events management.

TASK 4

You have been organising a modestly sized, open-air rock concert, but find your plans have been thrown into confusion by the impact of the ISE guidelines controversy.

Prepare a presentation, by which you would hope to persuade representatives of the ISE to abandon or modify their guidelines for an event such as yours. Point out the difficulties you would encounter in complying with their guidelines. You would also need to convince them of your ability to care for the health, safety and security of the public and your employees, without the benefit of the services of a chartered engineer.

Now that you are aware of the scope of health, safety and security legislation in the leisure and tourism industry, it is hoped this task may lead to broader discussions about the impact of the law, and where the balance might be found between the preservation of personal freedom and the need to protect the interests of the employee and the consumer.

CHECKLIST OF PORTFOLIO EVIDENCE

☑ Presentation

Glossary

Code of practice: part of the duties of the HSE is to issue codes of practice, explaining and further refining the Acts and regulations that govern the matter of health and safety at work. They have no legal status as such, but to disregard their recommendations is a failure that can be used as evidence in court should a prosecution occur.

EEC/EU directive: the directives of the European Union (formerly European Economic Community) are pieces of draft legislation intended to be taken into national law by the member states, in order to standardise the legal system across the Union. Although agreed by every state at European level, some contentious items can cause political problems at home. Delay or refusal to implement directives can be challenged by individuals through the European Court.

Health and Safety Commission: unlike the Executive, the Commission is a small panel used by the Department of Trade and Industry to consider matters of general policy in health and safety at work, and to report to the Secretary of State.

Health and Safety Executive (HSE): the HSE, whose powers derive from the Health and Safety at Work Act (1974), employs many hundreds of people at regional offices all over Britain and has responsibility for: enforcing health and safety legislation, inspecting workplaces, producing codes of practice and collating and publishing statistics. Its equivalent in Northern Ireland is the Health and Safety Agency for Northern Ireland.

Legislation: the sum total of enacted laws, comprising both Acts of Parliament and statutory regulations.

Parliamentary Act: Acts of Parliament are items of legislation that have been proposed, discussed, debated and finally voted on across the chambers and committee rooms of the Houses of Parliament. The passage of an Act is a lengthy process, so many are in part *enabling* measures, whose content give power to government ministers to issue further regulations without additional recourse to Parliament.

Personal protective equipment (PPE): many workers now routinely use items of PPE, such as chain-saw gauntlets, ear defenders and hard-hats. Their use is required by certain statutory regulations, which, together with codes of practice, should be consulted in all potentially hazardous situations.

Statutory regulations: these are items of legislation issued directly by government ministers, under the authority of enabling Acts of Parliament. They have proved a convenient way of empowering the many directives that arise from our membership of the European Union.

Visual display unit (VDU): cathode-ray tube television screens, commonly used on computers or wordprocessors. VDUs are common not only in the office workstation, but are also in places as diverse as the factory floor equipment control panel, airport check-in and entertainment lounge. Requirements for controlling the emission of radiation and other hazards associated with VDUs are covered by a statutory regulation and a code of practice.

Index